I0100510

Consistently Compassionate

Consistently Compassionate

Cali Mayne

Cali Mayne

Contents

Contents

III

Mindfulness

IV

Relationship with Self

V

Conclusion

Introduction

An estimated 50% of people quit a fitness program within 6 months of starting it, and over 40% of America's population is overweight according to the CDC.[1] Why can't we stick to a program and how can we keep obesity from rising? The answers are found in this book. Creating a sustainable lifestyle change does not come from having the perfect meal plan or workout routine but loving yourself enough to try again when things don't go as planned. Taking care of your physical health comes as a symptom of prioritizing your emotional health. Throughout this read, you will find advice covering nearly all aspects of wellness, including physical, mental, emotional, environmental, and spiritual health. As a human, none of your actions are independent of another, each aspect of life influences the others.

Fitness programs often fail because most personal trainers are advanced fitness enthusiasts. They've been doing this for years and are usually programming from their own experience. I know what it's like to have no idea what a "lat pulldown" is and thinking it kinda sounds like a dance move. Most people emphasize too much on getting results *fast* instead of making them *last* (just call me Dr. Seuss). Life is not a race. It's a journey.

You're going to have this body for the rest of your life, so becoming healthier will require creating some healthier habits. I know, you have trouble keeping those right? I did too. Then I started slow, making one small promise I could keep in under 10 minutes. I also started being nice to myself when I messed up, because what was the point in being mean? I was going to wake up with my consequences the next day, and I wanted to love myself enough to try again. And I want that for you, too. :) Also, we're humans, and we're bound to fail. No one is perfect, even though some people try to appear that way with their curated social media platforms. (I know you're struggling too Patricia; no one really knows what we're doing on this ball of confusion).

I want to help you believe in yourself enough to know you can achieve the life of your dreams. I plan to do this by providing education on nutrition, movement, and mindfulness, sharing personal *journal entries* that document how I was truly feeling throughout this process, and offering practical tips that have helped me along the way. The past 2.5 years have been the most rewarding, uncomfortable experience of my life.

Most mornings now, I wake up excited to tackle the day ahead, which is not something I could have said two years ago, but personal growth helps you see a new perspective on life. It is not easy to change, but you are worth any goal you want to achieve. Typically, having a goal means reaching a new level you haven't achieved yet; this means you will need to do things you've never done before in order to achieve that goal. Prepare to be uncomfortable, because our brains do not like change, but not *too* uncomfortable. Life will never give you more than you can handle. Even if you feel like there is no light at the end of the tunnel in your current situation, there is hope for a better future. No emotions last forever. Whatever higher power you believe in can confirm this. If you weren't ready, you wouldn't have the opportunity. And if you weren't capable, you wouldn't have the desire. Anything is possible if you believe in yourself, and I believe in you.

Consistency and compassion are two topics I will discuss frequently throughout this book. Not to quote Michael Scott... but, "*Webster's Dictionary* defines," consistency as "the quality or fact of staying the same at different times." Consistency requires choosing yourself and your needs more often than not. It's okay if you don't know what your needs are yet. You will learn what they are as you spend time with yourself. Consistency is the most efficient way for humans to develop a new pattern or habit. Compassion means being **kind** and **understanding** in times of "failure," or as I like to say, things not going as expected. Self-compassion often requires looking at a situation from two different sides. Seeing where you can grow as well as seeing that you are worthy of life, exactly as you are.

In May 2020, I quit my corporate job to focus on changing the aspects of my life I could control. This was a difficult decision, and I was terrified to place that much faith in myself. I didn't have a lot of money saved up, but I knew if I didn't change, my life would end quicker than I wanted it to. I value my life over money and material things, so it ultimately was the best decision for me. I began by meditating, walking more, and *attempting* to eat less fast food. I emphasized "attempting" if you didn't catch that (I still ate a lot of fast food).

I've struggled with emotional eating since childhood, specifically fast food. Since my nervous system was chronically in the sympathetic "fight or flight" state, leaving me in survival mode, I severed the connection between mind and body, so I did not receive signals of satiety or feeling full and satisfied. I would eat until I was so full, my body was in pain, and the pain was all I could focus on, instead of my feelings. I realized this concept by becoming conscious to my behaviors. I had to recognize and *accept* what I was doing in order to change it. This required becoming aware and consistently reminding myself that I am worthy and whole exactly as I am, regardless of the aspects I wanted to change about myself. Like everyone, I had done things in my past I was not proud of, but those behaviors were done out of survival mode, because I needed to feel safe. To begin to love myself, the first step was to forgive myself for the choices I made while operating in survival mode.

Have you ever sent an email with the phrase "per my last email" knowing very well the information was already covered at some point in the thread? Throughout this book, if you see the phrase "per my last email" it's because I've repeated information from somewhere else in the book, which means it's probably pretty important, which means it *may* be helpful advice to take away from the section. Why that phrase, you ask? Because that phrase is a vibe, thank you for not judging me.

Your body is like a car. It comes with an owner's manual, but *you* must find it. I can give you some of the instructions because as humans, there are certain things we all have in common, but you'll have to do some work on your own to find the other parts of the manual. Don't worry, the only thing you have in life is **time** to figure this out.

I

Nutrition

{ 1 }

The Only Rule

Rule #1 in the owner's manual, your body operates via energy. The realization of this universal truth helped me make sense of the enigma of weight loss that had been confusing me thus far in life. So much about losing weight never made sense. On the most basic level, in terms of nutrition, the energy you consume is calories. If you want to lose weight, you **need** to be in a calorie deficit. A calorie deficit means exerting more energy (calories) than you intake, which is the **only** rule you must follow to see results. This means you don't *have* to exercise to lose weight, but it does help. Sorry to just lay it on you like that, but I'll do a lot of truth telling in this book, so I thought it best to throw you in the deep end early. I work at a swim school right now, so the puns are constantly in my head.

You can find the number of calories a food has listed on the nutrition label of a package. There is an example of what this looks like on consistentlycompassionate.com as well as a ton of other information. You could also download a calorie tracking app like MyFitnessPal or LoseIt! and use the barcode scanning feature. Tracking calories is a great first step to become **compassionately** aware of what you're eating (how much energy you're putting in your body).

Is there a certain amount of energy you should be consuming every day? Why yes, yes there is. This is your Basal Metabolic Rate (BMR). Your BMR is the number of calories your body *needs* to continue automatic processes in the body like creating cells, processing food, maintaining body temperature, and keeping you happy, not hangry. This is based on your age, gender, height, and weight. Now, your Total Daily Energy Expenditure (TDEE) is your BMR + the number of calories you typically burn from exercise or physical activity. There's a lot of sciencey talk here but stick with me.

For example, my current BMR (this will change as your weight changes) is 1,582 calories per day. This means I should be eating *at least* 1,582 calories per day. My current TDEE is 2,175 calories. So, to be in a calorie deficit, I need to consume between 1,582 calories and 2,174 calories per day. Having a range of calories to eat can help simplify nutrition. No need to stress yourself out counting how many almond slivers you can have to hit a specific calorie goal. This frees up some mental space to focus on the present moment.

Under the nutrition tab on consistentlycompassionate.com, there is a "Calorie Deficit" page. If you scroll all the way to the bottom, you'll find a link where you can determine your **estimated** BMR and TDEE through calculator.net, which will give you the range of calories you would want to eat if your goal is to lose weight. Please, *please*, *please* keep in mind these numbers are **estimates,** and it's important to listen to your body. You know yourself better than anyone, especially better than calculator.net. Progress looks different for everyone. If you're eating 5,000 calories a day right now, it will not be reasonable to drop to 2,000 calories overnight. You need to be realistic and **compassionate** with yourself. If you're still hungry after you've consumed all your **estimated** calories for the day, you should eat more food. Per my last email, **it is important to listen to your body**.

It's important to become compassionately aware of how many calories you're consuming. This helps you know what progress will look like, because progress looks different for everyone, so there is no need to compare your progress to others. One way to become aware of how many calories you're consuming is to keep a journal or use a calorie tracking app. Do not expect yourself to remember to log every meal and snack all the time. You are not perfect and were never meant to be. When you forget, move on. Tomorrow is a new day. The most important aspect here is that you don't give up and be nice to yourself when you don't do exactly what you planned because no one is perfect.

Okay, so we've talked about calories, but how do we consume calories? I know, I can hear you right now. From food, Cali, *duh*. Yes, but what is *in* food? Macronutrients are food substances your body requires in large amounts to supply energy. You know how cars need a battery, an engine, and a transmission? They are three major parts to a car. Well think of macronutrients like the three major energy sources your body needs to function. These nutrients are carbohydrates, protein, and lipids (fat). Eating the correct amount of each macronutrient is dependent on your needs. You are different than everyone else with unique goals and lifestyle choices. There is no "one size fits all" diet that will work for everyone.

Each type of macronutrient supplies the body with different forms of energy, so depending on the intensity of exercise, a specific kind of energy will be used. There is a lot of complex science behind the different energy systems. Trust me when I say, "**a lot of complex science**." *wipes sweat off forehead* The National Academy of Sports Medicine (NASM) states, "Carbohydrates are the main substrate used during moderate to high-intensity exercise, whereas fat is the predominate substrate used during lower-intensity exercise." This means if you are exercising at a low intensity, your body (machine) is using the fat in your body to produce your movement. I am a *huge* advocate for low intensity exercise for many reasons.

1. If you are new to exercise, your body is not used to moving at high intensities. And if you attempt to work at high intensity, your body will likely be confused and not happy.
2. Low-intensity exercise has lower risk for injuries.
3. Walking is one of the most underrated forms of exercise.
4. Less sweat.

Okay, so just as important as the engine, transmission, and battery, cars also have all those little nuts, bolts and screws. For your body, these are micronutrients. Micronutrients are vitamins and minerals that your body needs for bodily processes. Each micronutrient plays an important role in your body. You can learn more about what each one does on consistentlycompassionate.com. Some vitamin and mineral deficiencies can play a part in physiological symptoms such as depression, fatigue, low energy, and irritability. It may not be your boss making you irritable, you could just be lacking B12 (It could also be your boss, idk). If you have the opportunity or availability to get tested for vitamin/mineral deficiencies I would highly recommend it, so you can ensure your machine has all of its nuts and bolts (I've been known to have a couple of screws loose occasionally).

Now that you know vitamins and minerals are essential to your body, it's important you keep them coming in. Eating a whole food diet is typically the best approach to ensure you're getting the proper nutrients. I know what you're thinking. *Duh, but I like chicken nuggets* (and same). You will not eat a whole food diet all the time. It is not feasible, and *very* few people actually do it. So, I like to supplement with a multivitamin, just to be sure.

Some vitamins are water-soluble, which means they can only be processed by water. This means you must hydrate!!!! Water is the most important compound for your body and an essential component for many bodily processes, like digestion, lubricating joints, and keeping your temperature regulated. Your body is 50-70% water. This is not a revolutionary thought but keeping water with you at all times will help you stay hydrated, and having a glass of water on your nightstand will help you stay hydrated throughout the night.

Imagine if you didn't put an oil filter on your car when you changed the oil.... That would be a disaster because it would obstruct your engine. For your body, this is what would happen if you didn't chew your food. Mastication (chewing) is a very important initiator of digestion. Proper chewing allows your body to easily break down nutrients once you swallow. Eating slowly, with little to no distractions, will help you to feel the cues of fullness. I don't know about you, but I never used to pay attention to how much I chewed. I would literally grab like five or six French fries at a time and *inhale* them. I used food to cope with emotions I was feeling, so eating quickly, without paying attention to how much I chewed, was a natural feeling. Learning the importance of chewing properly initially made me feel like I was dumb for not knowing that I should have been chewing more and slowing down when I was eating, but after being compassionate to myself and realizing that there was nothing wrong with who I was, that knowledge helped me enjoy smaller portions while still appreciating the taste of food.

Consistently Compassionate

It's okay that I used to eat like this! I did what made me happy and what I was familiar with. I ate French fries nearly every day for much of my life. It's what I grew up with and what I was used to. There is nothing wrong with that, but I wanted to live a healthier life. It's okay to have conflicting emotions about a situation. When I started this journey in May 2020, I ate a lot of fast food, especially when I was craving it. That was all I ate some days.

When I learned that a calorie deficit was the only rule I needed to follow to reach my goals AND that a Chick Fil A 8-count nugget is ONLY 270 calories, you bet your happy ass I was getting my nuggs. This experience also taught me I didn't have to get a value meal every time I went out to eat. I used to get a 12-count nugget meal, large, with a sweet tea, but tracking calories taught me I could order just enough food to fill me up.

Mindfulness (we will cover later), helped me realize when my body was not happy with my choices. Being aware of how my body was feeling made it hard to ignore the symptoms I felt from eating processed and greasy food. Don't get me wrong, in the moment, I was happy as could be. But later, when I was on the toilet or lethargic and sweaty, I couldn't help but notice how that food made my body feel (not great). I forgave myself and simply noticed how my body reacted to the decisions I made regarding what kind of fuel I put in the tank (another car reference). Since I wanted to be kind to myself, I began *wanting* to eat foods that made my body feel good and perform at its most efficient.

<u>December 2020</u>

> *I went to Chick Fil A for lunch because I genuinely wanted it, my body was feeling good, and I was craving it, so I went to get it. After work, I went to the gym, then went out of town to go Christmas shopping. On the way home, I passed one of my favorite fast-food places, Sonic, and I was like "Ooooh, I want that." But then I was like, "stop, think about what your body is actually feeling right now." My body does not feel good. My stomach hurts, and it's prob from the Chick Fil A earlier, so I'm not sure if my mind releases serotonin* [not serotonin, dopamine, but hey, I'm proud of myself for thinking it was a chemical!] *when I eat fast food, which is maybe why my brain was like "Ooooh I want that Sonic" but I know my body does not want that right now.*

Speaking of noticing how my body feels, one morning in July 2021, my stomach started growling. And I thought, "Okay, I hear you, thank you for letting me know I need food." Which is definitely not something I would have said to myself before. This was a dramatic shift to what I used to experience. Before this mindset shift, especially when I was younger, I would wake up with hunger pains, wanting to eat almost immediately, and I felt so much shame and guilt around those experiences.

But who I was during that time was exactly where I was meant to be. If I would not have experienced that, I would not have this comparison. Just like who *you* are right now is exactly who you are meant to be. Accepting yourself as you are, will be the key to change. There is absolutely nothing wrong with who you are, *especially* not because of the amount or type of food you eat.

Per my last email, a whole food diet is the healthiest way to intake the necessary nutrients to make our bodies run the most efficiently. **However, life is not all about efficiency.** Life is experiencing love, joy, memory making, efficiency, convenience, and many other things. If it were feasible to eat a whole food diet 100% of the time, everyone would do it, but it's not. And very, very, *very* few people do it. That's why I initially took the 80/20 approach. Moderation is key for this approach. 80% of the time, I would **try** to eat a whole food diet, while the other 20% of the time, I indulged in the foods that bring me joy regardless of their nutrient content. I eat chicken nuggets on a regular basis. It's my favorite food.

Most of the time now, I enjoy the taste of healthy foods

because they taste like being able to get out of bed without pain. They taste like the warm sun on my skin while hiking through the woods. They taste like freedom and better quality of life. Being compassionate around food for me looked like the journal entries below.

<u>January 2021</u>

> *I don't feel like a failure because I fell "off track" because it's not really falling off track. I had an issue with my family, and I still haven't recovered from what happened. I'm still emotionally wounded by it. But I needed to take time to heal those wounds, so I focused more of my energy on that instead of exercising, specifically. My nutrition has still been relatively on point but there were a few changes. Since it's the holidays, I was gifted cupcakes and chocolate. 1. It would be rude to turn them down and 2. This isn't an all or nothing mentality for me. I want to fix my relationship with food so that I can eat intuitively for the rest of my life to be happy and healthy. At the beginning of December 2020, I was 251 and at the beginning of January 2021, I was 257. Six pounds of regain does not make me a failure.*

<u>August 2021</u>

> *Today I am grateful for my self-compassion, because I know that no matter what happens tomorrow, I will be okay, #1 and #2 - I want to eat vegetables and proteins and things that make my body feel good, because I know I am worthy of that and my body is my vehicle, and I should put premium in it. I am grateful for being graceful with*

myself when I've messed up in the past so that I can learn the lessons that I needed to, to be where I am today.

Being consistently compassionate with myself helps me understand that no matter what has happened in my life, I'm not a bad person. I have only been experiencing what life has put in front of me and doing the best that I can with what I have. This goes for everyone. Being nice to myself felt odd and uncomfortable at the beginning. I was so used to letting my brain tell me that I was unworthy of my life. I heard voices in my head saying I wasn't good enough for love or even to live. Actively deciding those voices were wrong, changed the way I looked at myself. Practicing gratitude has allowed me to see the prosperity I already have. Being poor doesn't come from having too little but from wanting more. Recognizing your abundance means realizing what you can *do* with what you already have.

{ 3 }

Practical Applications for Your Abundance

This chapter will entail some real-world advice on how to heal your relationship with food, a journal entry template to practice daily change, and some recipes on how you can incorporate some new foods into your life (don't be scared to try new things).

Digestible (pun intended) advice on how to improve your relationship with food:

- Forgive yourself when you eat something you didn't *actually* want to eat. Even if, when you ate it, you were happy with your choice in the moment.
- Accept the fact that progress happens in many forms. If you ate 5,000 calories yesterday. Eating 4,500 calories today is progress. And forgive yourself when you don't progress. You won't make progress every day, and that's okay.

- Shift your mindset of physiological cues of hunger (stomach growling, thoughts about food, poor concentration). They occur to help you, not shame you. Accept them with kindness and use them as a guide to make decisions on when to fuel your body.
- Eat mindfully by limiting distractions and paying attention to how much you chew. Mastication (chewing) is an important process for the digestive system. *Practice* noticing how long and often you chew.
- Keep water with you as often as possible. Just having water around will be a helpful reminder to stay hydrated. You could designate a cup holder in your car to your water bottle or keep a spot available on your nightstand.

One of Dr. Nicole LePera's tools is called the Future Self Journal. Below is an example of part of one I did. Feel free to use this as a template to create your own. Writing down your goals will bring you closer to achieving them.

October 2020

- *What pattern or behavior do I want to change?*
    - *I want to improve my relationship with food.*
- *Statements that will help me achieve this:*
    - *My body deserves to be nourished.*
    - *I am grateful to eat because food makes me stronger.*
    - *Even if I overate yesterday, I still need to eat today.*

- ◦ *My size does not define my health.*
- ◦ *I am in tune with my body and respect my hunger cues.*
- ◦ *I choose to be at peace with and be kind to my body.*
- *How will you practice these new behaviors in daily life?*
  - ◦ *I will listen to my body for signs of hunger.*
  - ◦ *I will increase water intake.*

Recipe for Most Efficient Meal Prep (MEMP) - Makes 4 Meals

<u>What you need:</u>
Microwave
Oven
Baking sheet
Cooking spray
1 package of chicken tenderloins (6-9 pieces)
Bag of frozen vegetables (your choice)
4 Individual microwaveable rice cups
Seasoning (your choice)

<u>Directions:</u>
Preheat oven to 385°F
Get out a baking sheet and coat it with cooking spray
Clean and place chicken tenderloins on sheet and season
Once oven is preheated, place in oven for 17 minutes
(internal temperature should be 165°F to be cooked thoroughly)

While chicken is baking, put bag of frozen vegetables in microwave for recommended time (mine is usually 6 minutes)

While vegetables are microwaving, get out your meal prep containers.

Once vegetables are finished, take them out and set them aside.

Now, start microwaving individual serving cups of rice, one at a time.

Begin portioning the veggies & season while the rice cups are still microwaving.

Once all the rice cups have been microwaved, portion into containers.

By this time, the chicken should be finished, take out of oven and check temperature.

Allow the chicken to cool, then portion into containers.

Recipe for Veggie Delight – Makes 1 Serving

<u>What you need:</u>
Stove
Cutting board
Knife
Medium to large saucepan
Stirring utensil
Butter or cooking spray to coat the pan
2 tablespoons of butter
1 medium Zucchini

Consistently Compassionate

1 medium Tomato
1 tablespoon of cream cheese
2 tablespoon parmesan
Salt
Pepper
Italian seasoning
Fresh basil (optional)

Directions:
Cut zucchini into small pieces
Coat the bottom of the medium saucepan with butter or cooking spray and turn burner on medium to low heat
Place zucchini in saucepan to sauté, season with salt, pepper, and Italian seasoning – should take about 10 minutes, depending on how small you cut the pieces
While zucchini is sauteing, cut tomato into smaller pieces (size doesn't matter too much here because it will cook down anyway to turn into a sauce of sorts)
Once zucchini begins to darken with signs of being cooked, add 1 tablespoon of butter, and cut tomatoes into saucepan
Reduce heat to low and stir
Allow to simmer and cook down for about 7 minutes, stirring occasionally
Add cream cheese, parmesan, and basil (optional) stirring to combine
Let cool and enjoy!

Optionally, you could serve this over rice or pasta.

CALI MAYNE

{ 4 }

Be Yourself – The Right People Will Gravitate

We've all heard this advice, right? You're stressed about a project at school or a big presentation at work. You go to a friend, partner, or parent for support, and what do they say? Just be yourself. While this is solid advice, it implies we know who we are. Being yourself is one of the biggest tasks you will undertake in this lifetime. Many of us are still not aware that we even have our own individual personalities and interests. Well, at least I didn't know until about the age of 23. Get to know yourself. Learning who you are and remaining true to that standard may shift where you are in life, but it will bring new people your way, ones that will love you for you, unconditionally.

If you don't like chicken, rice, or vegetables (you might want to try some new vegetables), please don't use the meal prep offered in the last chapter. Being yourself in terms of nutrition, means eating foods *you* enjoy. No one can tell you what those are. This is part of the owner's manual you must figure out on your own. This will require trial and error with new foods. When I was 25 years old, I figured out I love cucumbers. The last time I tried one before 25, I was 9. Since my palate wasn't used to raw vegetables, I thought it was disgusting, lol. Are we surprised? Watching thousands of people's "What I Eat in a Day" on Instagram, YouTube, Facebook or TikTok may be super helpful to get inspiration, but if you don't like the food they're eating, don't make it. When you go to the produce and meat section, what sparks your interest? Do you like bananas? Do you like apples? Do you like oranges? Broccoli? Peaches? Carrots? These will be the foods you'll want to start incorporating in your diet. If you don't like what you prepare, you won't eat it. I know you know what I mean. Aunt Petunia always brings macaroni salad to the BBQ, but you don't like it, so you swerve past, polite as possible, while asking about her husband who's gone a lot because he drives an 18-wheeler? You know what I mean.

If you don't normally shop in the produce section, it's normal to feel uncomfortable going there the first couple of times. No one is looking at you and no one knows it's your first time there. You deserve to take up space in that section, just like any other human. If you don't normally get produce, don't overwhelm yourself. Only try one new thing. The next time you come back, maybe you'll try two items!

The internet has a vast number of meal ideas and recipes. We live in an age where literally anything you want to know can be found at your fingertips. Use this to your benefit, not your detriment. Recipes shouldn't be complicated or take a lot of time. You don't want to put a lot of effort into making nutrition complicated. Making new decisions and changing your behaviors will be hard enough. You should try to keep nutrition and movement as simple as possible. Most of my meals are relatively boring to other people, but for me, I get to eat my favorite foods constantly.

Also, be yourself when it comes to how you want to track your calories. Per my last email, becoming aware of how many calories you're eating is going to be a huge first step to becoming healthier. Get an idea of the number of calories you consume, in whatever way that works for you. You could keep a physical notebook or notes in your phone and jot down how many calories are in a food before you eat it. Forgive yourself when you don't record your calories every day. We are humans, we are not perfect. You don't have to share this with anyone unless you feel comfortable doing so. It doesn't have to make sense to anyone other than you.

It was difficult for me to begin tracking my calories. I didn't want anyone to know how much food I ate on a daily basis. I always felt ashamed. Deep down, I knew what I was doing wasn't healthy for me, but I felt stuck, in a constant loop of betraying myself and what I truly wanted. My experience with nutrition may likely sound similar to yours.

My Experience with Nutrition

One of my caregivers always used to tell me, "All you have to do is cut out fast food, and you'll lose weight." I finally realized what worked for her didn't necessarily work for me because I needed to get to the root of the problem. Throughout my childhood, I didn't learn much about proper nutrition or how to fuel my body for movement. Since my caretakers were constantly stressed with work and raising two children, many of our meals came from drive-throughs. I don't blame my parents. They were doing the best they could with the knowledge and resources they had. There wasn't a lot of apparent evidence, **available to everyone**, regarding the poor quality of processed food, and at the time, all the benefits seemed to outweigh any perceived negatives. Fast food appears quick, easy, and cheap.

When I was 17, the summer before my senior year of high school, I, unsustainably, lost about 50 pounds from fat burners and being *extremely* rigid with my diet, not allowing myself to indulge at all. I remember one of my volleyball teammates saying, "Wow, Cali, you look amazing." This filled my heart with joy. I really felt like I had done something amazing, but I hadn't eaten any "cheat foods" (I don't use this term anymore because all foods can fit in a well-balanced diet) throughout the entire summer. Then, our coaches ordered pizza one day after school. My teammates were enjoying their food, and I remember the conflict in my mind because I wanted the pizza, but I knew I was going to relapse or go back into my old habit of overeating hyperpalatable foods like fats, sugars and salts. "One slice won't hurt, Cali," My friends lovingly encouraged me. I know their intentions were pure, but they did not understand the decision I had to make. Back into the cycle I went.

Because our brains oppose change, we typically take habits from childhood into adulthood, and I was no exception. Most days in college, I would have Burger King for breakfast (a sausage, egg, and cheese croissant meal, sometimes 2 sandwiches if I was really hungry). For lunch, I would either get Dairy Queen (Chicken tender meal with a sundae to dip my fries in) or McDonalds (Large 10-piece chicken nugget meal with a sweet tea) and on the way home from work I would get either DQ or Mickey D's, whichever I didn't have for lunch because they were right next to each other.

I remember having arguments in my head when passing fast-food restaurants about whether or not I needed to stop. Sometimes, I would use the traffic light for justification. There's a Chick Fil A on the left side of the highway in my town. If the left arrow was green, I would think to myself "It's okay to get it because the light is green. The universe is giving me a sign," I told myself. I began to think I was crazy and trapped in this constant cycle. If you also struggle with these internal arguments, you are not alone and there is hope for change. Start by recognizing these conversations are okay. There is nothing wrong with who you are.

I personally began tracking calories through the Lose It! App. The barcode scanner made the process so easy and convenient, because when I started to pay attention to what I ate, most of the foods were prepackaged, which makes sense, because I didn't know how to cook much of anything.

Starting to track my calories allowed me to become aware of how many calories were in the foods I ate consistently (270 calories for an 8-count Chick Fil A nuggs). Once I started to get a feel for checking calories prior to eating something, I stopped meticulously tracking because it didn't make me happy, and I was still seeing progress without doing it. Everyone is different. The key here is that I was honest and compassionate with myself.

I didn't know how to cook very well, but over time I learned, and I'm still learning today. I have some meals that are staples, and I can throw together quickly because I've made them so many times (MEMP). Below is a journal entry from one of the best "wins" I've had with my relationship with food. Keep in mind, I didn't like salad for the first 25 years of my life.

-
October 2021

> *I've never had Zaxby's before. So, I wanted to try it. I pulled up to the menu and I was like meh, none of this looks appetizing. Then I saw a southwest salad they had, and I was like, that looks good. *shock* I'm sorry what? From the girl who used to eat chicken nuggets and French fries for every meal of the day? She wants a salad from a place that specializes in chicken? And the lady was like, do you want grilled or fried? And I said grilled without even thinking about it."*

Nutrition is a key component of the human experience. Without food, we would not survive. I met a woman once who explained how she felt about food. She understood that she uses food to cope with reality just as other humans use drugs, alcohol, or shopping. She said something along the lines of, "Using food to cope sucks because you can't get away from it. If you smoke or drink, you can just stop buying cigarettes or alcohol, but food is necessary." This is why healing your relationship with food is essential for sustainable weight loss.

Another aspect of human existence is movement. This is not something we could completely eradicate, and if we tried, we would begin to decay. Movement is necessary for the body and mind to function properly. There must be balance though, right? If your body is not used to moving quickly and intensely every day, that would be a jarring change for your being. Movement can come in many shapes and forms. Let's dive a little deeper.

II

Movement

{ 6 }

VT1 & NEAT

Just like a car needs to move or the battery will drain, our bodies like to move every day. If you're just beginning to move your body regularly, you should do it every day (as often as possible but be kind to yourself when you don't). The more consistently you move, even if it's for a short period of time, you are building a habit. Also, the more often you do it, the more times you can learn from the experience. This means you may experience some feedback, like feeling excitement from doing specific activities (walking, dancing, stretching, yoga, swimming or any other movement activity you can think of that you would enjoy). This feedback can help you determine which activities you'd like to continue pursuing.

You may be thinking, but what about all the jacked people who go to the gym 3 times a week for 2 hours? Well, they have different goals than you. They are likely building muscle, which requires rest between muscle-building days. It's okay to have different goals than others, even if you aspire to look like them. Some people were born with bodily/kinesthetic intelligence which is one type of intelligence that means being able to feel your muscles as you move. If you were not born with a strong sense of this ability, it will take time to develop it. So, if you cannot feel your muscles individually, you are not alone, but if you trust the process long enough, you will be able to feel your body as a machine. You will begin to feel your hamstrings contract as you walk.

Increasing this intelligence will increase the amount of awareness you have around your body. It will also build your relationship with yourself because you will be able to take cues and feedback if your body is sending you signals. Don't worry if you don't have a lot of points in this stat though, you were born with other types of intelligences, that other people may not be very strong in. We're all born with different stats in different types of intelligence; there are nine types. You can find them here: https://www.consistentlycompassionate.com/whoareyou

-

December 2021 & January 2022

> *I stretched my hip flexors consistently for 3 months and I can start to feel them when I'm walking (12.31.21) allowing me to adjust my gait (1.1.22) I ADJUSTED MY OWN GAIT.*

Some general benefits of movement are listed below:

- Improved ability to do daily activities
- Reduced anxiety

- Increased chances of living longer
- Reduced depression
- Increased fall prevention
- Increased positive mood
- Reduced risk of some cancers
- Improved self-esteem
- Reduced health risk of cardiovascular disease
- Improved cognitive function
- Weight management
- Alleviated symptoms of social withdrawal
- Better quality of sleep
- Reduced risk of type 2 diabetes
- Strengthened bones and muscles
- Improved overall quality of life

Let's talk about some aspects of movement that are important for your body. Low-intensity movement, Ventilatory Threshold 1 (VT1), flexibility, and Non-Exercise Activity Thermogenesis (NEAT), which can be described as a fancy way of doing daily activities that are not sedentary. It is pretty neat lol. Per my last email, your body will primarily use fat as the energy source during low-intensity exercise. I'm going to explain *a little bit* of the science to help you determine if the rate you're going is still considered low intensity.

As you're exercising, when you increase the intensity of your body moving, more oxygen is needed to keep up with producing more energy. This will cause you to breathe heavier to intake more oxygen. Once you begin to struggle having a conversation while moving, you have likely switched into VT1 which is when lactate begins to accumulate in the blood, so your body is using an equal mix of fats and carbo-hydrates as the energy source. Basically, when you're moving your body, keep it light enough to where you can continue a conversation, and your body will be using fat as the main source of energy. This is important because each person will have their own VT1.

This means going on a walk and having a conversation with your best friend is a perfect way to exercise. While you're walking and talking, practice active listening and calming your mind. You can also take time to look at nature and the beauty all around you. Practice hearing what your friend says and try to imagine how you would feel in their shoes. Don't try to relate to an experience you've had, really listen. Don't think about how you'll respond while they're talking. When they've finished is when you can pause and choose how you want to respond. Slow down. Life is not a race. I doubt your friend will be impatient for a response from you.

Flexibility is the range of motion of your joints or the ability of your joints to move freely. Doing flexibility train-ing can increase your range of motion and reduce the risk of injuries. Also, this kind of training is *usually* low intensity. Flexibility training is one of the most practical forms of ex-ercise. You can stand almost anywhere and start stretching. I used to do posture stretches *frequently* while working at Planet Fitness Winchester.

Non-Exercise Activity Thermogenesis (NEAT) is a drawn-out way of saying "using energy to do daily activities other than planned exercise." This is doing activities like walking your dog, getting the mail from the mailbox, walking from your car into the house, making dinner, or pretty much any movement you do other than being sedentary (sitting or lying down). Increasing NEAT will allow you to burn more calories without even realizing it.

<u>Practical applications to help increase flexibility and NEAT</u>

- When storing items in your house, place the most used items just out of reach so you can stretch muscles you don't normally stretch. (If you choose to try this, please don't make it too hard on yourself, *just* out of reach).
- Listening to music while doing chores will help move your body more.
- While hanging out with friends or family in a comfortable location, you can get on the floor and stretch. Please note, if you try this and your company is not accepting or encouraging of this, you may want to evaluate this relationship. Don't be afraid to set boundaries. This is your life. How they react to your boundaries is none of your business. It is better to have a view than to be viewed (credit to Alexis Craig for that gem of a phrase).
- If you live within walking distance of any errands,

use your feet instead of your car. Save gas and the environment. :)

- Park at the back of the parking lot to increase steps.
- Whenever you remember to do it: engage your core/"drawing in maneuver" (PT language)/"make yourself skinny" (that's how I knew to do that motion as a kid).

Now that you know what aspects of movement are important, don't forget to be kind to yourself when you don't incorporate these newfound lessons. Change is an overwhelming task for the ego to comprehend. Slowly, but consistently adding new ideas and tasks into your life, while remaining compassionate with yourself, will create a sustainable lifestyle change.

{ 7 }

Consistently Compassionate

When I first started to engage my core, I remember thinking, "How is this going to help? I only remember to do it for like 30 seconds when I'm on a walk." But then I started to do it for 45 seconds, then a minute, now I remember to do it for more than half of my walks and sometimes when I'm performing exercises. I'm still growing and learning every day.

When I started moving my body in May 2020, I was in my bedroom, trying different activities I thought I might like. I did a lot of dance cardio - it was incredibly fun, and I looked absolutely ridiculous, but I heard someone say once, "If you can't be cheesy, you can't be free." I was also doing 6-minute strength workouts, because I couldn't bring my body to move any more than that (and that's okay), but I was instilling a habit. The main difference on why I used to fail versus why I've been consistent this time, is because I've been compassionate with myself when 6 minutes of movement was all I could do. Our society has depicted perfectionism as if it's real. No one is perfect and you should never be unkind to yourself when you don't achieve perfection because it does not exist.

If you are just beginning to move your body regularly, how can you expect yourself to do the same things as someone who has been doing this for years? If you're just starting to change your habits, every workout will not feel great. Most days, I didn't even feel the muscles I was supposed to be working. But I trusted myself and the process. You should always strive for success, but don't give up because your workout isn't absolutely amazing every time.

You will get to the point when you're performing an exercise, and it'll click. You will feel the correct muscle group contract and elongate as you perform the exercise. Trusting yourself and the process is extremely rewarding. Do your best to be present (more on this in the mindfulness section) during your movement activity. Try to keep your core engaged and focus on what muscles you're supposed to be working.

December 2020

> *My workout felt great tonight. I did core and back. Also snagged a pic of flexed back for a b4 pic later. :b So excited w/ the physical progress I'm making, but the most exciting progress personally is my codependency. I'm finally*

learning to tune into my physical body & understand that my emotions & body regulations are just as, if not more important than anyone around me.

No one will do this for you. It's entirely up to you to make the decision to change your habits, but that doesn't mean you have to do it alone. Having a social support group can be extremely helpful. The best place to look for people who share your goals is where you pursue those goals. I was reflecting on getting a gym membership in this journal entry:

<u>November 2020</u>

I think one of the most daunting things about starting a workout routine is that we feel like we have to know what we're doing all the time. Although it's nice to have a plan, it's not always necessary. I'm thinking about getting a gym membership because it's getting cold af outside. I was feeling nervous because there are a lot of options at the gym, but then I thought, "Why are you going to be nervous? You're gonna walk on the treadmill at the gym because you walk outside right now. Don't overthink it.

You may not always have the same support system though. Not everyone in your life will choose to take the same path as you, and that's okay. Keep choosing yourself. Life will bring the right people to you.

<u>October 2021</u>

One of the toughest lessons I've learned so far is that the people who are in your life that you love very much, do not also have to change their lives. And if they don't, you feel less connected to them, less relatable. It's very sad, feeling like you're no longer understood by the people who have been with you for a long time. And if you're not good at making new friends, you don't really get to find new people to love right away.

<u>Ways I was consistent and compassionate with myself around movement throughout my journey:</u>

- Forgiving myself when I left the gym early without completing my entire workout routine because I didn't have the energy.
- Getting home late, still doing a leg workout and walking a mile in the house because I had the energy to.
- Doing an arm workout at home while listening to "I'll Be" by Edwin McCain, crying in the middle of the work out because of how proud I was of myself for getting to where I was, then finishing my workout while watching my favorite musical (Phantom of the Opera).
- Recognizing when I was struggling with my self-worth, acknowledging those feelings as neither good nor bad, and making a plan to get back on track with my movement goals by journaling.

Okay so, we know that we can move our bodies slowly, while still making progress. We also know to be kind to our bodies and ourselves when we don't do exactly as we planned, because sometimes, things don't go as expected. Let's talk about posture. This is the fundamental base of your movement style. This is often overlooked, but is essential to proper form and safe movement.

8

Posture

Posture is the foundation of how your body functions. If your posture is not allowing your body to move the most efficiently, this should be the first thing you work on. You don't have to spend a lot of time on your posture every day. I started out spending two minutes a day on my posture with the YWTL stretch. I found this series of four stretches through a chiropractor on YouTube. The Y looks like you're doing the Y from the YMCA dance. W looks like you're a football referee declaring a field goal. T looks like a scarecrow in the middle of a field. L looks like the opposite of W, instead of having your hands pointed up, they would be pointed down (you can find a video on www.consistently-compassionate.com).

Standing up straight and engaging your core (when you remember to do it, which will not be all the time) will help you recognize your power that you can achieve anything. One way to improve confidence is by correcting your posture. I can tell as I walk around that people look at me more now than they used to because I carry an energy of self-respect. Confidence is one of the most attractive things a person can display.

In the following journal entry, I describe how I felt when I really struggled with my body image regarding my posture. I remember standing in the women's workout room in Gold's Gym, feeling my internal body temperature rise, my hands sweating, and my face flush red. I felt so embarrassed, like there was nothing I could do to help myself. *Now*, we know that's not true, but at the time, I felt so scared and alone. I wanted someone to fix me or save me, but I'm the only person who can do that, and I reminded myself that no emotion lasts forever.

July 2021

> *Today has not been good for me. I almost walked out of the gym after realizing how bad my body is. I have muscular imbalances everywhere. My posture is so bad, but I can do anything. I can fix my posture and make my muscle mass bigger. I can do it. It's going to take a lot of time, but I can do it.*

With proper posture, the risk of injury is reduced, and movement can be performed more efficiently. According to NASM, there are three postural distortions that many Americans struggle with due to the modern American lifestyle. These patterns produce muscle imbalances which cause our bodies to distort from its most functional form. Muscle imbalances occur when certain muscles are working harder than their counterparts. Consequently, some muscles are overactive, and some are underactive. You can correct this by strengthening the underactive muscles and stretching the overactive muscles.

I've created a stretch routine for overactive muscles affected by the three distortion patterns. This routine should take no longer than 15 minutes to complete. I have done this routine *almost* every day (because humans aren't perfect) since August 2021 to help improve my posture. If you choose to try this routine, hold each pose for 30 seconds, if you can. For the YWTL, keep your thumbs pointed behind you, pinch your shoulder blades together and engage your core. For all the stretches, try to remember to keep your core engaged. You won't remember to do it for every stretch and every time and that's okay! I'm so proud of you.

One of the simplest ways you can take care of your body is to focus on how you're treating it in this moment. Focusing on your posture by engaging your core and standing up straight will not only boost your confidence, but also create a happy, healthy body for your soul to live in. If you can remember to do it occasionally, that's awesome. If you want to set a reminder on your phone, that's cool too. Find what works for you and run with it. You're not supposed to be anyone other than you.

9

Be Yourself – The Right Activities Will Come

It's also okay if you don't want to stretch. Stretching is an activity that will help you gain more flexibility and increase your range of motion, but if you don't care about that stuff, don't do it. In order to remain consistent with movement, you need to move your body in ways you enjoy, or you will not stick to it. Does that sound familiar? This journey is about **you**.

Finding what you enjoy will require trial and error. This may also require being uncomfortable. When you try new things, your brain is very wary, which makes your body feel uncomfortable. If you start to do something you know will be beneficial and you hear a voice saying, "It's not enough, this little bit isn't going to help." That voice is not correct. Anything extra you do will not hurt; it will only help.

You may think you like doing an activity, then get half-way through and be like, "Nah, this aint it, chief." And that's okay. You can always try something new until you find what you enjoy or if you felt a spark of excitement, try that activity again to see if the uncomfortable feeling goes away the next couple of times. The movement you choose to do may not be traditional, but if you're moving your body, you **are** making progress, regardless of what anyone has to say about it. Believe in yourself to make the best decision for you. Remember, it doesn't have to make sense to anyone else, only you.

"Out of the box" movement ideas:

- Dancing around the house
- Rollerblading
- Play tag with family/friends
- Swimming
- Live Action Role Playing (LARPing)
- Paintball
- Quidditch ;)

I've become confident with movement because I know my goals are not the same as those around me, so if I'm moving my body differently than someone else, it doesn't mean I'm doing something wrong. This means we are different people with goals based on our own needs. I enjoy walking like a model on the treadmill, so I blast "Bezos I" by Bo Burnham and strut my stuff. Which is probably why I used to find myself in the cardio cinema at Gold's Gym a lot, but now I do it in public, idc. After going to a new gym to try it out, I wrote the journal entry below. It's safe to say I really learned something about myself that day.

April 2021

> _I love moving my body, but I like it when I do it by myself. And I'm okay with that. It is okay to want to be alone. It's okay to want to do things by yourself. It has taken me a long time to learn that I'm not a socialite. I don't have to be social. I think that's what I was so lost on. I felt like I had to be social, I had to go meet people, I had to go to the gym if I want to be in shape. But I don't. I bought three dumbbells and I've been doing home workouts with them._

The key here is to spend some time with yourself and discover what you enjoy. Spending time and enjoying the presence of others is important but there must be a balance. Finding time to meet your true self will help you discover who you truly want to be. My experience with movement has evolved rapidly as I've discovered my true Self.

10

My Experience with Movement

I've been moving my body pretty frequently since child-hood. Starting at 4 years old, I did cheerleading, gymnas-tics, and baseball. In middle school, I played volleyball and basketball. During my 7th grade basketball season, I scored 4 points the whole season, and both shots happened in the last game. I was the "MVP," let me tell you. (Also, I had to be taken out of the game right after I made the second shot because I was winded af). In high school, I played softball and volleyball.

In the last journal entry I reflected on the fact that I don't enjoy being social often. This may seem like a contra-diction to all the team sports I played throughout childhood. Well, that's because it is. When I realized I enjoy move-ment in solitude, I had recognized, accepted, and overcome some codependency, which can be described as emotional or psychological dependence on someone else. (See Appendix A for more information). As a child and young adult, I felt as though I was not worthy of love if I didn't accomplish things that made my parents proud. This typically showed up as making the sports team or getting good grades. I was not living for myself.

In no way, shape, or form do I blame my parents now. When I first learned about codependency and **trauma**, did I hold some resentment? Of course. This was a very natural and human emotion I needed to work through, and it took me about a year to get through it. If you share this experience, it may take more or less time for you to work through these feelings. Honor your experience; it will be different than everyone else's. Trauma is an experience of energy that occurs within the body when the Self has been suppressed.

Once I realized my caregivers were doing the best they could with what they had, I felt compassion for them. This is how they were raised. They were treated the same way when they were children. They were not encouraged to find their unique abilities, but to sacrifice their own needs for love too. This is a common form of trauma (See Appendix B for more information) humans experience. And to be fair, they didn't have the internet, therapy wasn't accessible, and in my family (like many others), therapy holds a stigma.

After learning I enjoy solitary movement activities, I began exploring nature. Walking and hiking are two activities I enjoy very much because I can incorporate aspects of life I love. Typically, when I'm walking, I move like a model and listen to music because that makes me feel confident and sexy. When I'm hiking, I get to see nature. I love watching animals and seeing different kinds of trees.

<u>Ways that movement has specifically benefitted me:</u>

- Being flexible enough to bring my foot close enough to my hands to clip my toenails.
- Being able to tell my family that I was going for a jog when I've **never** said anything like that before.
- Being able to cross my legs.
- Being flexible enough to shave comfortably (huge win).
- Walking to my job (at the time) instead of driving, saving time at the gym and money in gas.
- Being able to adjust my gait (manner of walking, pace/stride length), by consistently stretching my hip flexors.
- Being grateful for the tree that provided shade every time I took a break from work to go stretch.

Movement plays a key role the overall health of our bodies. Creating a movement routine that *you* enjoy is essential to creating a sustainable habit. If my experience with movement has resonated with you in any way, you likely struggle with a disconnection between your mind and body, like I did. One way to heal this disconnect is through mindfulness.

III

Mindfulness

(Reminder: If you cannot be cheesy, you cannot be free)
Mindfulness is being consciously aware of your surroundings, behaviors, thoughts, and feelings. Once you accept the fact that the only thing you can control is the way you react to situations, you will have the power to take control of your life.

I know what you're probably thinking. "Cali, this book is supposed to be about weight loss." This is much more than just weight loss. This will help you create a lifestyle change so you can live the life of your dreams. That's why there's more information than just nutrition. Because if it was just about weight loss, you would only need to know that you must be in a calorie deficit. This could've been a pretty short book, but you *deserve* to know how I made this change and how it could be possible for you.

{ **11** }

Meditation & Nervous System Activations

"Meditation practice isn't about trying to throw ourselves away and become something better. It's about
befriending who we are already." – Pema Chödrön

Do you ever feel like you just can't keep your brain quiet?
Are thoughts of the past, missed opportunities, and regrets
are so much louder than everything else going on around
you? Would you like to shed your racing thoughts, anxiety,
and judgement of yourself? If you answered yes to any of
these questions, go ahead and take two *deep* breaths from the
belly, really expand your stomach. Each time you're inhaling,
think about how your body feels when you're inhaling. Then,
when you're exhaling, think about how it feels to exhale.
Close your eyes if you'd like. Go ahead... How did that feel?
If it felt good and you want to keep going, set a timer for 30
seconds and do it until the timer sounds.

Meditation is an ancient practice that helps you become aware of your physical body and allows you to observe your thoughts. Recognizing that your thoughts are not who you *are* but simply ideas that come and go within your mind will allow you to watch them change instead of letting them dictate your behavior.

Thoughts will constantly come into your mind. Focusing solely on your physical body in the present moment will allow you to recognize *when* thoughts are entering your mind. This will take time to develop. Meditation will likely feel uncomfortable the first couple of times you do it. Remember: trying new things feels uncomfortable. Your brain likes familiar.

The practice of meditation is recognizing when a thought is arising. You probably won't realize when a thought enters your mind immediately. You may entertain it all the way through its process, but when you become aware, you can make a mental note of "thinking." Sometimes it's helpful to say it aloud. Being aware of your thoughts allows you to approve what you want to say and do instead of reacting emotionally to your thoughts. When you love something, you don't judge it, right? With the absence of judgement, you can witness and accept your behavior to decide what you would like to change.

This may come as a shock to you, but I'm here to give you the truth. As a collective, we have the opportunity to evolve into a creative species, but within our society, most people are living in survival mode; constantly activating their sympathetic "fight or flight" nervous system (often not on purpose and completely unaware). When your sympathetic nervous system is activated, you don't feel safe in your body. You feel overwhelmed, out of control, or on edge. You believe the world is dangerous, threatening, or out to get you. When attempting to connect with others, you feel like authentic connection is impossible or you need to be defensive. Understandably so, because when this nervous system is activated, you may confuse neutral facial expressions as hostile.

When your parasympathetic "rest and digest" nervous system is activated, you feel at peace, relaxed and curious. The world feels safe, like it's not out to get you. With others, you can make eye contact, and vulnerability and trust become safe. During this state, it feels possible to manage life: you can make clear decisions and be creative (See Appendix C for more information).

If you didn't jump straight to the appendix to learn more, I *know* what you're thinking. HOW DO I ACTIVATE THE SECOND ONE? I ALWAYS WANNA BE IN THE SECOND ONE! The first step is to become a **witness** to your body, your experience, and how you are feeling. One way to practice this is: you guessed it, meditation (I always try to come full circle).

When you begin meditating, you will become aware of your body and you will become aware of your thoughts, so this means: You are not your body nor your mind, there is an essence within you that has a purpose here. You were given these assets to work for you, not against you. The universe wants to work in your favor as long as you follow your soul.

Keep this simple and easy. Allow yourself to be, however

you are. Reflect on how you're feeling and **sit with it**, instead of changing it, do not act, just sit with it. If you're sad, be sad. If you're angry, be angry. If you're joyful, be joyful. If you're confused, lost, or scared, allow these feelings. All emotions are temporary. Remind yourself of this when you're feeling emotions that are not ideal. You are a complex being with a huge range of emotions. You should become familiar with all of them, not just the ones you're comfortable with. Below is a journal entry of a moment when I was conscious of my thoughts and feelings. I recognized I was anxious about a time that had not even arrived yet.

June 2021

> *Nothing bad (extremely jarring) will happen tomorrow. You can handle anything that comes at you. Unless you die (then you don't have to worry about it). Don't let your brain say you can't do something. You're incredible. You have no idea how much power you have. You can only control yourself. Everything else, let it be.*

These topics were hard for me to handle when I first learned about them. They added additional meaning to the life I thought was so simple before. Humans have so many layers, but when I boil everything down, one thing always remains: love. As long as I love myself and do what I need to do to truly meet my needs (feeding myself the proper macronutrients and micronutrients, moving my body, allowing my inner child to be free, healing my trauma), I am a better person than I once was, changing the world for the better.

CALI MAYNE

Consistently Compassionate

Mindfulness involves time spent alone with yourself. This can be uncomfortable if you feel shame or guilt around who you think you are. If you feel this way, you will come to understand that the person you currently are practices learned behaviors to keep you safe. You don't eat fast food every day because you think it tastes good. Your body is conditioned to believe it brings you happiness. Neuroplasticity is the concept that the way we think can be changed over time through experience (Appendix E). By rewiring your synaptic connections in the brain, typically through experience, this can change.

I recently learned about a term called "anti-fat bias." The National Academy of Sports Medicine (NASM)[2] states this as "placing a negative judgement on overweight or obese individuals." Let me tell you, when I read that, my heart sank. I finally had a term and understanding for why I used to feel the way I did about myself. I used to feel so much shame for the way I looked.

I've been overweight since I was a child. I know my shame was conditioned. There is absolutely nothing wrong with who you are. Society has glorified thin people and demonized (harsh word but feels true) those who are overweight. If you are overweight and were raised with anti-fat bias in your household, I am giving you a big hug right now. I'm so proud of you, and it's finally time to put that heavy burden down. You are so beautiful exactly as you are.

Being compassionate regarding mindfulness, for me, sounded like talking to myself. A lot. I remember asking, "Why are you so upset with yourself for not knowing how to do something you've never given yourself the chance to learn?" It also sounded like, "Sometimes, I want someone to appreciate how much I've grown in the past couple of years, as much as I know I deserve to be appreciated, but then I remember, that's what *I'm* here for."

I used to tell myself that I couldn't read books because I didn't like to be alone with my thoughts, and that was *so* real. I didn't like who I was, so I didn't think nice things about myself. It was hard to learn anything new with consistent thoughts of self-loathing running through my mind. I don't think I was alone in that. I think a lot of humans' experience feelings of shame and guilt around who they are.

You deserve kindness and compassion. You are whole and worthy, exactly as you are. Once you accept yourself for who you are, all your individuality and uniqueness, you will open the doors of possibility so you can transform into who you truly want to be. This is the first step to *real* change. This life is yours to live, and you can do anything humanly possible.

While I whole-heartedly agree that self-discipline is the key to achieving goals, when I first started this journey, I did not have the confidence or self-efficacy to even think of self-discipline as a concept. So, if you're anything like I was—you don't like yourself and changing doesn't even sound possible —try accepting yourself as you are right now and loving yourself first. Once you begin to consistently treat yourself with compassion, you will crave self-discipline because you know you are worth it.

Practical ways I began to love myself:

- Becoming a witness and recognizing when negative thoughts about myself arose and allowing them to pass without dwelling on them or judging them.
- Looking in the mirror often! I finally learned to appreciate that I am a human being with my own feelings and needs.
- Writing positive affirmations on mirrors/locations I look every day.
- Reflecting on situations that didn't work out the way I expected with an open mind (ex. What can I learn from this?)
- Practice releasing expectations of others, unless I share a close relationship with them that allows for *healthy* expectations (this could be a whole 'nother book).

- Forgiving myself when I make decisions that don't align with my goals.

The coolest part (IMO) of learning to love myself is giving each interaction I have with someone, everything I have, because if that person is meant to be in my life, they will receive the love I'm emitting and reciprocate the same energy. If they are not meant to be in my life, they will not. When I interact with someone, I'm being my authentic self because I finally love her, and she's allowed out. This means the right people will come into my life because I'm not pretending to be someone I'm not. I'm not ashamed of my quirky laugh or the fact that I enjoy skipping. Yes, I skip often. Sometimes at work. Mostly on the way to my car though. Here are some particularly compassionate feelings for myself during a meditation session.

September 2021

> This morning during meditation I felt like I was receding in progress. My mind was wandering far more often than it had been, and then I realized that I am going through an entirely different situation than I had been in the past couple of months, and I gave myself grace once my mind started to wander. I began again, focusing on the breath each time. Knowing I am not giving up is the best feeling in the world.

Asking someone to love themselves if they haven't done

so in the past is a huge task to overcome. It may take months or years to adjust to this new mindset. Often when we're being our own biggest critics, we're comparing our experience to someone around us, thinking that we're not good enough. But on the contrary, we are exactly where we're supposed to be.

{ 13 }

Comparison

"Comparison is the thief of joy." – Theodore Roosevelt.

As you know, all humans are unique individuals with specific talents and traits to share. Accepting this fact will allow you to break free from the chains of comparison because no other person shares your journey or experience. I usually find myself comparing a lot when I'm in the gym or doing physical activities. Instead of focusing on performing at 100%, I look at those around me, simply viewing them as bodies, forgetting they have their own personal lives with challenges to overcome too.

One thing I've never struggled with is being competent at a job, I can easily (usually) follow directions and complete tasks as asked. That is not something everyone has the capability of doing. I'm also rather skilled at being a mediator and helping people see points of view other than their own. Remembering that I have different skillsets, helps me focus on the challenges I must overcome instead of comparing one aspect of my life to one aspect of another human's life.

Comparing yourself to someone who has different skills and struggles than you will not benefit you in any way (See Appendix D for more information). This is one reason why mindfulness is so important. It allows you to be one with yourself where you can learn who *you* are, instead of relying on the current aspects of your personality to determine who you think you are.

From a young age, I compared myself to my sister who happens to have a smaller body frame than I do. I idolized her. She was exactly what I wanted to look like. I remember taking her clothes because I thought wearing them would make me look like her, but I kinda sorta just stretched them out... sorry Cass.

When I was in high school, I was told I didn't make the varsity softball team because I was overweight. Instead of looking at the situation as, "This extra weight is prohibiting me from being efficient enough to compete properly," I compared myself to the girls who happened to have a smaller body frame, but who *could* perform efficiently enough to compete on the varsity team. At the time I felt hurt, like I would never be good enough as long as I was overweight. After reflecting on the situation, I know the decision had nothing to do with my worth and everything to do with my performance.

I believe the majority of society looks down on people who are overweight, but not for the reason I initially thought. It has nothing to do with the inherent worthiness of the person, but the capability to manage life. Having extra weight and fat in the body can be a detriment to one's physical health and makes managing life more difficult.

I tried to lose weight so many times in the past with the comparison mindset. I would look at models and celebrities who lost weight, and I felt so shameful. If they can do it, why can't I? That mindset never worked out because I didn't care if I ate poorly, was lazy, or felt lethargic. I expected my life to remain the same, and I would magically become thin. I wanted to lose weight so that I could feel worthy and be respected by others, but that's not how life works. You have to respect yourself before others will truly respect you.

There will always be someone who is "prettier," "smarter" "wealthier" or "snazzier" than you, as long as you see it that way. To quote Qveen Herby, "What good is being fly, in someone else's eyes?" We will all thrive and succeed once we begin to understand ourselves. The only person you should compare yourself to is the yesterday version of you. Because it will always be you vs you. This journal entry came from a proud moment when I began to focus on the most important comparison: current me vs. past me.

January 2021

I'm watching Meet the Robinsons right now. I was thinking about my weight loss progress since January and all I can think of is "Keep Moving Forward." Just keep moving forward, one day at a time. Win small battles every day.

Consistently Compassionate

In a lecture on "The Art of Being Yourself," Caroline McHugh discusses three ways of being in the world: superior, inferior, and interior. If you have a superiority complex, you believe you are better than others. An inferiority complex implies you are less than others or that someone needs to find you out. But an interiority complex means you simply belong and you deserve to take up space, just like everyone around you. It's completely uncomparative. We all have the right to be comfortable with who we are. Releasing the thoughts of being better or less than anyone else can free up so much mental space. Allowing you to be more mindful of the present moment.

{ 14 }

Benefits of Mindfulness

Mindfulness seems like a lot of work for little reward, right? Think again. There are physical, mental, and spiritual benefits to mindfulness. All for the low cost of putting aside time to spend with yourself in silence and practicing witnessing your thoughts as thoughts, not reality. One thing I've noticed when I observe people around me is that there usually seems to be some sort of distraction. It may be another person, a phone, TV, or even a book. Although any form of media and distraction can be beneficial in moderation, I rarely see humans sitting in silence, with themselves. And if they are, it may be that thoughts have taken over. Meditation is the act of witnessing your thoughts and finding peace in silence. Once you become an observer of your thoughts, you can gain the benefits of mindfulness or rather, release all that worries you.

A physical benefit of mindfulness is the mind-muscle connection. Remember bodily/kinesthetic intelligence? This can be described as feeling the muscles in your body during movement. You may be thinking, *So wait, Cali, you're telling me I can practice this outside of the gym?* Freaking cool, right? After spending so much time in the gym, I no longer have a routine (other than my stretching routine). I've strengthened the mind-muscle connection so much, when I walk in the gym, I let my body tell *me* what needs to be worked on that day. Talk about clearing up some mental space.

Being mindful of your body can also help you heal trauma stuck in the body (See Appendix E for more information). When trauma, an event of energy that occurs within the body when the Self has been suppressed, happens, it can cause physiological symptoms such as headaches, sweaty palms, racing heart, hunched posture, and stomach pains. When you experience trauma, you sever the connection between your body and mind so you may not even be aware of these physiological symptoms at times. Some ways to heal trauma stuck in the body are stretching, placing attention on certain areas of the body and conscious, deep belly breathing.

Being aware of your body and its needs will help you communicate those needs with people around you, allowing you to show up as your genuine self. If you honor yourself by keeping promises to do things you enjoy, that spark excitement, and you feel compassion for yourself, you will teach other people how you want to be treated. For example, when I started going to the gym on a regular basis because I made that commitment to myself, my family just expected me to be at the gym. I showed up late for Christmas 2021 because I was (I'll give you three chances to guess where I was and the first two don't count) ... Yeah, I was at the gym, and no one even batted an eye. It became what they expected of me because I expected it of myself.

Some mental benefits include better sleep, more creativity, less anxiety and less depression. Falling asleep becomes easier because your thoughts are no longer in control. Your spirit begins to take this place. You can practice placing your attention in your body and drift effortlessly off to sleep. Once you practice realizing negative thoughts are just thoughts and that they don't dictate your life or actions, you can allow your inner child to escape and be creative by singing, dancing, painting, playing music and/or sharing your story with the world. We need you to do this. You will change the world for the better!

What if I told you your anxiety is just your "ability to focus" trying to determine the future? And what about depression? What if that is just your "ability to focus" stuck in the past? What would happen if you placed your attention, your focus, on the present moment? Would you be free from these thoughts?

One of the spiritual benefits of mindfulness for me was learning trauma I experienced and recognizing how it made me behave towards food. As a child, when I did not feel safe in my body, I would dissociate or go into dorsal vagal (Appendix B) or "shut down" mode and eat food until I couldn't feel anymore. Because I severed the connection between my mind and body, I didn't receive physiological cues for satiety or feelings of fullness and satisfaction. I remember mindlessly eating French fries and chicken nuggets until I couldn't stand how full I was. Below is a journal entry of how mindfulness and compassion shifted my perspective around hunger cues.

-

<u>October 2021</u>

> *During my meditation this morning my stomach growled. This was met with, "I hear you, I acknowledge you, thank you for letting me know that my body is hungry." In the past, that action would have been met with, "This is why we're fat. Why are you always hungry?"*

Mindfulness also helps you become aware of how you're feeling. One benefit of this is limiting social media to only those who bring you joy, push you to grow, and challenge you to learn new things. No more following people who post useless content that's irrelevant to your life or say things that make you feel like poop. This will allow you to keep your mindset focused on what is important to you. If you're following a fitness influencer who says things like "I had a cheat meal this weekend" or "If it's Monday and you didn't work out, you're garbage." How do they make you feel? You are what you consume, this includes social media, friendships, books, and food. Anything you spend time with will develop you as a person.

These benefits will not appear overnight. The only way to create a sustainable lifestyle change is through daily **practice.** Practice means pausing before you react or repeat the same behaviors. In order to practice mindfulness, it's imperative to pause before making a choice on how to react to a situation. To make a sustainable change in your life, your

lifestyle will change. One helpful tip to experience the benefits of mindfulness is to release the expectations of how you
think your life should turn out and embrace the good around
you at any given moment. This moment is the only thing we
truly have. There will always be good and bad in any situation, what you focus on is what your life will be. I used to
focus on the negatives constantly, until I learned that life is
perspective, influencing my experience with mindfulness.

{ 15 }

My Experience with Mindfulness

I remember doing the dishes one morning, probably about 4 years ago. I was about halfway through, and I was thinking "Yes! I haven't felt resentful towards Tim for not doing his dishes before he went to bed." Then, boom, I started having resentful thoughts, which I then took out on him when he woke up later that morning. Looking back on that situation now, I realize I could have **paused**, recognized that thought as just that, a thought, and went on with my day.

Recently I came home to visit because I've spent the past two months living and working on a farm, and I'm grateful to have the opportunity to take care of some stray dishes in the sink. Life is perspective. It's not about what happens to you, it's about how you react to it.

As a teenager and young adult, I thought about death almost every day. I used to think about suicide often because I truly believed I was not worthy of my life. When I read the phrase, "if you were not worthy of life, it would not be," my world was changed. I began to prioritize my mental, physical, and spiritual health, and some relationships started to dissolve. This was painful to accept at first, but then I realized anyone who has my best interest at heart would stick around through all my phases, even if it's at a distance.

In 2020, I was 25 years old waking up with zero motivation to get out of bed. I felt like my life was already over. My body fat percentage was over 50%, I had chest pains, poor-quality sleep, and was winded *often*. Mindfulness encouraged me to recognize my behaviors and *slowly* change my habits over time. Per my last email, one of Dr. LePera's tools is called the Future Self Journal. This can be extremely helpful in creating new habits. Below is an example of part of one I did.

October 2020

- *Daily affirmation:*
    - *I am my own person who has emotions.*
- *Today I focused shifting my pattern of:*
    - *Dependence on others*
- *I am grateful for:*
    - *Having no physical disabilities*
- *3 traits my future self will have are:*
    - *Emotional independence*
    - *Societal comfort*
    - *Will power*
- *The person I'm becoming will experience more:*

  ◦ *Confidence*
• *I have an opportunity to be my future self today by:*
  ◦ *Setting boundaries*
• *When I think about the person I'm becoming I feel:*
  ◦ *Peaceful*

One of my biggest influences on social media is Dr. Nicole Lepera. She posts as @The.Holisitic.Psychologist on Instagram and has written *How to Do the Work*. Dr. LePera has also created the SelfHealers Circle, which is an online community, and the SelfHealers Soundboard podcast where she and Jenna Weakland discuss Dr. LePera's book and other topics regarding holistic psychology and practical tips on "how to do the work" of healing. Her content is extremely cut and dry. She makes learning *how* to heal very simple, not that healing itself is simple because it's individualized. In my humble opinion, she is truly changing the world. One of the first concepts she approaches in her book is consciousness – how to recognize behavior, accept it and change what you can control.

I was working at Walmart in December of 2017. Oof, what a way to start a story, but stay with me. I remember going outside because I was so overwhelmed with emotions and thoughts. I felt like I couldn't control myself, and I was going to start crying. I didn't want to break down in that store (again) or be controlled by my emotions, so I sat on the edge of a parking space, cross-legged, bundled up in a sweatshirt. As I sat there, I remembered reading something about "just focus on your breath." So that's what I did. I inhaled and thought solely about how it felt to inhale, then I exhaled and thought solely about how it felt to exhale, probably for about 15 seconds. After that night, I didn't seriously attempt meditation for another couple of years, but I do remember having the **courage** to try something new that night.

In February of 2021, I started working as an office assistant, so I could listen to music, audiobooks, or podcasts while I worked. It was a reeeeeally sweet gig. I stumbled across a podcast called Ten Percent Happier, where they discuss ways to become (you guessed it) 10% happier. And honestly, who doesn't want to be happier? Meditation is a recurring topic on that podcast, so I decided to give it another shot.

I began meditating for 1–2-minutes at a time, until I realized I wanted more time calming my mind. So, I slowly progressed from 5 minutes to 10 minutes. Today, I meditate for about 15 minutes every morning and it helps me feel more present throughout the day. Sometimes I will find a quick moment during the day to tune into my body if I'm feeling particularly overwhelmed with thoughts by taking a couple of deep belly breaths and focusing on the inhale and exhale. When unhelpful or negative thoughts arise, I allow them to come and go because I know that no emotion lasts forever.

I used to feel very disconnected from other humans, as though they would never understand me. Through mindfulness, I learned, this feeling was because I felt disconnected from myself, and I did not validate my own experience as a human. I would often look in the mirror and feel numb. I did not accept myself as a person with my own feelings and choices. As a human, you are never alone because you always have yourself. Whenever you are feeling lonely, ask yourself "what do I need?"

Mindfulness wins for me sounded like having conversations with my ego (self-talk in the mind, the thoughts that arise to help keep you safe). Being aware of my ego and accepting it as it is allows me to create positive thoughts like, "I'm doing well," and "I see you trying your best." My ego says things like, "I'm not good enough" and "I'll never be anything successful." My ego is only trying to keep me safe, so I welcome the thought, allow it to speak its peace, and wait for it to exit. The more I practice creating positive thoughts, the stronger that pathway becomes in my mind. This is an example of neuroplasticity. (See Appendix F for more information).

Ways to practice mindfulness:

- Meditation: there are guided meditation videos on YouTube.
- Conscious breathing exercises: I have used the Breathwrk app.
- Mind-muscle connection during movement: look in the mirror to see your muscle, take deep breaths and drop in to how your body is feeling, engage your core whenever you remember to do it.
- Journaling: old fashioned paper and pen work best for me but notes on your phone could be just as helpful.
- Eating with no distractions.
- Connecting to silence: feeling what your body feels

like with no distractions present, similar to meditation. Silence may feel unsafe to some people, so it's important to become aware of your relationship with silence and slowly begin to incorporate it.

My experience with mindfulness has been an ever-evolving journey that began with a 15 second meditation in a Walmart parking lot. After practicing meditation over the years, I've come to realize a few things. As a species, we are all made up of the same elements, meaning we are all the same. Whatever created this existence lives within us. We are all gods in our own right. Meaning the relationship with yourself will determine the relationship you have with life. The microcosm reflects the macrocosm. Healing the relationship with yourself will create the capability to heal the world around you. Love energy is the key to a meaningful life.

IV

Relationship with Self

It is said you can search the entire universe for some-one who is more deserving of your love and affection than you are, and you won't find that person anywhere. The most important relationship you have is the one with yourself. This sets the tone for every other relationship. The way you show up in the world and the role you play in others' lives is a direct reflection of how you feel about yourself.

Spending time with myself was extremely uncomfortable at first. Per my last email, I didn't like myself. I know I'm not the only person who feels this way. Do you struggle to *authentically* connect with others? Do you find yourself judging others when they're talking to you? Whatever you're judging them for, these are things you need to accept within yourself.

{ **16** }

Resilience & Confidence

As you make mistakes in life, you have one of two choices. You can dwell on the error, tell yourself you will never be good enough to complete the task and give up entirely. OR you can recognize making mistakes is a part of life, reflect on what can be done differently next time to avoid said mistake, and move on with your day. Consistently choosing the latter allows for growth. Now, I know what you're thinking... *Easier said than done, Cali.* And you're right, it's *much* easier said than done. You probably have negative thought patterns instilled in your mind from childhood, but just as the negative thoughts were taught, positive or compassionate thoughts can be established instead. Remember, through experience, the way we think can be changed over time and with **practice**.

The journal entry below describes a time when I was sitting in my car on lunch break from work. In this moment, I had rapid thoughts of worthlessness because I deeply believed I had to be perfect, and what I was feeling in that moment was simply not good enough.

<u>*September 2021*</u>

> *My thoughts of worthlessness and just giving up are so strong today. I am such a good person; I deserve to be alive. I deserve to be happy. I deserve to be at peace. I just want someone to save me, but I know no one can. I can only save myself, but this is so hard.*

As I type these words, I struggle to believe I can write this book. These days will happen in life. Regardless of how much you've grown or changed, life is a cycle of new challenges. These cycles teach resilience and confidence. Encountering struggles to overcome creates a greater capacity for what you can handle in the future. Life will never give you more than you can handle, so after a struggle has been overcome, confidence is soon to follow.

<u>*August 2021*</u>

> *Life will never go your way 100% of the time. Even if you try to be the best person you can be and try not to harm anyone, life will never give you what you want all of the time. The only thing I want right now is to talk to someone and feel heard and validated. Sometimes it can be lonely. But that's okay because I know that this moment is only going to make me stronger.*

Resilience requires being okay with not being perfect and accepting that rejection is only protection from things that weren't meant for you, even if you wanted it. It means understanding that life will undoubtedly give you challenges and to expect the unexpected, or maybe to release your expectations. Amor Fati is a Latin phrase meaning "love of fate." This idea pairs well with resilience because it means that no matter what has happened to you, it's really happening for you. If something happens unexpectedly, life is trying to teach you something. Overcoming the challenge is what creates resilience.

Confidence for me looked like trying on bathing suits the night before I went to a new gym with a pool and feeling proud of the way I looked in each outfit. It also manifested in taking the practice Certified Personal Trainer (CPT) exam before looking at any of the content and being proud of my result, which happened to be a 54%. I technically failed, *but* I remembered this was just a practice test. I still had the opportunity to learn the content and take more practice tests before I took the final exam. Being consistently compassionate with yourself may not be easy, and it may be because you have experienced trauma (see Appendix B), which makes you believe you are not worthy of praise without sacrificing your needs for love.

You may struggle with negative self-talk and lack of self-efficacy, like I do/did. For me, this was displayed in the forms of self-betrayal, lack of trust in myself and others, and codependency (see Appendix A) by people pleasing. Creating a compassionate relationship with yourself opens doors for the possibility of change and growth because you love yourself enough to try, fail, and try again.

Choosing to be compassionate toward yourself does not mean denying negative experiences, it means *embracing* them. Understanding that every situation is temporary and even negative experiences have lessons within them, can help you learn from all situations. Although life may not have happened as you expected, there is something you can learn from every situation. Taking responsibility for your role in your life will allow you to learn from unexpected circumstances. The more you choose to see the good in who you are and what you experience, the more you open yourself up to transformation. Loving yourself isn't a selfish act but an act of self-acceptance. Choosing to be more compassionate around what you experience will allow you to have more peace, be more confident in yourself, and trust yourself. This may sound like telling yourself:

- "I can do this."
- "I will get through this period of my life."
- "This is temporary, no emotion last forever."
- "Look how far I've come."
- "I am proud of doing this even though I am scared."
- "I'm allowed to take up space and feel joy."

From a young age, you were taught that making mistakes is not a good thing, when the truth is, to err is human and the only way to grow and learn is by "failing" and trying again. Perfectionism is not real. You are a human, and you were born to make mistakes. There is no such thing as "failure" if you keep trying. Did you "fail" because you didn't get the outcome you wanted? Why? What happened that you could change for next time when you try again?

Learning how to change things to work for you is vital to success. Every human will have their own form of self-care because we're all individual creatures with our own talents and gifts to share. Two plus two equals four but three plus one also equals four. Just because your neighbor puts their trash out the evening before the sanitation service comes doesn't mean you have to. As long as you get it out before they come in the morning, the same task was achieved. It's important to discover who you are so you can be yourself.

Be Yourself

When you were born, you were gifted special talents and abilities that allow you to fulfill your destiny on Earth. Typically, we are not encouraged to discover these gifts, but to fall in line with a path that may be more logical or safe. You are not meant to be like those around you. You are supposed to be different. There will only ever be one "you," so it's important to take time to discover who you are and what you enjoy. The things that excite you are not random, they are aligned with your purpose. Recognize what makes your soul feel alive and continue to do those things. Can you remember the last time you had chills? This is your body giving you a sign that you enjoy what is happening. Follow these signs. Whoever you want to be, own it. No one needs to approve, except you.

<u>Ways to improve your relationship with yourself:</u>

- Determine your values. What do you think is important in your life?
- If you don't feel like you're living for yourself but to make other people happy, learn about codependency. (I read *How to Do the Work* by Dr. Nicole LePera, see Appendix G).
- If you feel like you're living for yourself but are not sure what you like to do yet, focus on the aspects of your life when you feel total joy. This would be when you're in a flow state. Recognizing when you feel this way may help you find your passion. If you never find yourself in this state, you may struggle with self-regulating your emotions (See Appendix H for more information).
- Be proud of yourself when you do something that aligns with your goals. Celebrate even the smallest of achievements but be sure to celebrate in ways *you* enjoy.
- Do a self-audit – write down any goals you have. Examine them to make sure they're what will truly make you happy. If not, you may not be living for your highest potential.

Working at Planet Fitness Winchester was one of the most thought-provoking times of my life. I found a group of people who accepted me for exactly who I was but challenged me to learn new perspectives and expand my skillset. After I spent time with myself, and learned more about who I was, I started doing things that sparked excitement for me but may have seemed "odd" to others. If it was nice outside during my lunch break, I would eat standing behind my car while dancing and singing. This was one way to "be myself." I also became open-minded and curious in conversations. I had one conversation with a coworker that changed my life. Below is the journal entry from that day.

October 2021

> *Today was one of the best days I've had in months for sure. I had a conversation with someone that has changed my life. This person asked me questions that I've never been asked before. They made me feel like I wasn't crazy for thinking the things I think. Put yourself out there, BE REAL. Humans are so relatable because we all feel the same things. Some feel them more than others. Anyway, this person gave me hope that I will meet other people in my future that won't think my mindset is a burden, that it's not exhausting to have a conversation with me. It makes me feel like I'm not alone. And that's really all I can ask for.*

Once you begin to learn who you truly are, release expectations of what other people think of you, and peel back all the coping behaviors you learned to keep you safe, you will find this pure essence who is joyful, curious, creative, and loving. This soul wants to explore and be free. Finding your soul will feel like death. In order to make room for your soul, you must grieve your past self. This can feel extremely lonely and scary. No one will know exactly how you're feeling, but there are people who have experienced this transition within themselves. You can certainly reach out to me if you ever would like to talk. You are never alone.

When you begin to learn who you are and love yourself, you will start to build your reputation with yourself. You will begin to keep promises to yourself and trust your intuition on what moves to make next in life.

{ 18 }

Trust Yourself

To learn to trust yourself, begin keeping one **small** promise a day that takes under 10 minutes to complete. Keep this promise every day (as often as you can and be kind to yourself when you don't) until it becomes a habit. For example, if you want to begin moving your body more, do a movement activity **you enjoy** every day for 10 minutes until it's a part of your routine. The habits I initially started forming were meditation, walking, and drinking more water. Trusting myself has also looked like (some of these were extremely scary):

- Going multiple days without tracking calories and still making progress.
- Doing yoga alone in a crowded gym.
- Ending a 5-year relationship.
- Leaving jobs because they did not align with my values.
- Choosing to eat food that other people called "unhealthy" because I know my body is different than theirs.

• Writing this book. I am doing everything in my power to trust myself. Being courageous allows you to level up in life (Super Mario sound).

Once I strengthened the compassionate mindset where I truly believed I could achieve my goals, I began to trust myself. I started with trusting my judgement on what foods I ate and the way I moved my body. I knew I could make the right decisions for myself, whether they made sense to anyone else or not. Trusting yourself can be difficult if you have previously sacrificed your needs to gain love or if you have consistently betrayed your own trust

From my experience, honesty is a rare trait in adults, but if you can find the courage to be honest with yourself, you may achieve your wildest dreams. This includes being honest about the way you feel. It doesn't necessarily mean you have to share it with others, but you at least need to be honest with yourself about how your life is going. Are you happy with all aspects of your life? If you're reading this, I would say probably not. In order to actually change, it's imperative to be honest with yourself regarding the role you play in your own life.

Blaming anyone else for the problems in your life will only keep you stuck in that constant victim loop. Because they are your problems, only you can solve them. Even if that means changing your perspective of what constitutes a "problem." It's time to call yourself out, but remember, the past version of you deserves compassion. If we turned back time, you would still make that decision. You did the best you could, with the knowledge you had, because you didn't know then, what you know now. It's unfair of you to use information and experience you've learned after the fact to judge yourself for decisions you've made in the past. Be true to yourself and trust the timing of your life. You are exactly where you are supposed to be (see Appendix C). You know yourself better than anyone knows you.

Since we are all the creators of our own life, we know what will work best for us when solving a problem, but I like to use something called discernment. This means I try to take the opportunity to learn from anyone and anything around me but trust myself enough to only *use* what works for me. For example, if I'm doing a task at work and someone approaches me with their preferred way to do said task, I will listen to what they have to say, try it for myself, and if it works better than how I was doing it, cool! I found a more efficient way to complete the task (with the help of said coworker) but if the way I was doing it is more efficient for me, I thank them for their advice and continue to do it my way. 1 + 3 = 4 just like 2 + 2 = 4. There are multiple ways to find solutions to problems. Trust yourself to find the best solution for your problem but be open-minded enough to try new possibilities.

Trusting myself felt very overwhelming at first. I was questioning every decision I made. Since I used to betray my own trust so often, it felt like I was living a completely different life. Remember, trying new things feels uncomfortable, so when I began keeping promises to myself, my ego did not like it. Change is weird for humans. My experience with Self has been a whirlwind of highs and lows.

From a young age, I felt shame about my size because most people around me praised and appreciated smaller body types, as I'm sure you can understand. This is trauma (see Appendix B) I need to heal from. When I was in 4th grade, I decided I wanted to be a teacher. This made my mom extremely proud, and since I learned to sacrifice my needs for love, that's who I was until the college semester before student teaching. Around this time, I began to learn about codependency (see Appendix A) and started making decisions I felt were right for me. After I changed majors, I felt lost and confused, unsure of what I wanted to do with my life.

When I graduated from college, I was still working at Walmart, so I decided to look for an office job. I found work as an admissions representative for an online university. This was my first "big girl job." I had no idea what I was doing, but I quickly discovered that most humans don't quite know what they're doing. We're all just trying to figure out life, same as the next guy. So, I started learning about myself. I took personality tests and noticed what activities made me truly joyful.

I realized I enjoy learning about human behavior and philosophy, so I delved into information around those topics. I started following social media accounts that provided information I thought was fascinating. I also learned I didn't think I was beautiful or worthy of my life. How did I figure this out? Becoming conscious of my behaviors, I realized I told my boyfriend, "You are not allowed to propose to me until I'm skinny." What a statement... I can't imagine how confused he was because I also got frustrated when he never proposed. Like come on Cali, pick a side...

My initial goal was to lose weight, but after learning *why* I didn't feel beautiful, my goals changed. Now, my goals are to fix my relationship with food, get stronger, feel better, and have more energy. After discovering my ability to be compassionate with myself, I knew I could change my habits to reverse the consequences of my previous behaviors. And so can you.

As I began to uncover the coping behaviors I exhibited to keep me safe, I found this pure, childlike essence that loves all humans and feels whole without the approval of others. A few of my coping behaviors were as follows: emotionally reactive eating hyperpalatable foods to cope with reality, making fun of my weight to mask feelings of insecurity about my body shape, and spending money on unnecessary material objects to fill a void because I thought that's what life was about. These were learned behaviors and all behaviors use energy. It took time and money to go buy food or to go to the store to shop. These habits were replaced with learning to cook and going to the gym. There are 24 hours in the day, regardless of which activities you choose to do. I sleep much better and have more energy throughout the day now that I have adjusted the behaviors I exhibit.

V

Conclusion

Just like a caterpillar, you have the opportunity to transform into the person you truly want to be. But the caterpillar is already something to be celebrated and accepted, and **so are you**. In order to transform, you must accept yourself as you are. Become a witness to your behavior and give yourself compassion. Past, present, and future you deserve this because you are doing the best you can with the tools you have. The four key concepts I've discussed throughout this book are nutrition, movement, mindfulness, and relationship with Self. Each one plays a vital role in the human experience.

Nutrition is an essential part of maintaining your body's efficiency. Macro- and micronutrients are building blocks to bodily processes and provide energy. Understanding and implementing a calorie deficit while including the foods **you** enjoy, will be a huge first step to lose unwanted weight.

Movement has many benefits of the mind and body. You have a variety of options to find what type of movement

you enjoy best and improving your posture will be a game changer for confidence and overall quality of life.

Mindfulness facilitates awareness around your behaviors and decisions. This allows **you** to witness who you currently are while encouraging you to stay present.

Exposing the soul within you by peeling back the layers of learned behaviors will allow **you** to meet your true Self. Having a consistently compassionate and positive relationship with yourself, will allow you to create opportunities for change and growth.

I believe my purpose in life is to share my story. I have overcome emotional eating and severe lack of self-worth (which I still struggle with some days) to bring you this book. My mission is to create an impact on the world by offering an alternative strategy to love yourself through education on nutrition, movement, mindfulness, Self-discovery, and consistent self-compassion.

Remember, this is about you. Accepting yourself for exactly who you are right now, learning what you enjoy, and trusting yourself to make the right decisions for you, will be the key to transformation. I believe in you, and I love you.

Appendix & Endnotes

Appendix

Appendix A: Video of Dr. Nicole LePera explaining codependency which may help you determine if you're codependent. https://www.youtube.com/watch?v=VYsRF29V4F0&t=17s

Appendix B: Video on the expanded definition of trauma. https://www.youtube.com/watch?v=iNP6pSkmS6M

Appendix C: Video of how our nervous system affects us. https://www.youtube.com/watch?v=IhUaxgzWxnI&t=207s

Appendix D: Video on being exactly where you are meant to be. https://www.youtube.com/watch?v=HqYEWub1eno

Appendix E: Video on what trauma can look like in the body and how to heal it. https://www.youtube.com/watch?v=kSPqM_Kkqng

Appendix F: Short video on neuroplasticity and how you can rewire your brain. https://www.youtube.com/watch?v=ELpfYCZa87g

Appendix G: Link to learn more about *How to Do the Work* by Dr. Nicole LePera. https://theholisticpsychologist.com/book/

Appendix H: Video on how to self-regulate: the ability to direct thoughts, emotions, and behaviors. https://www.youtube.com/watch?v=NxrfDovnjA4

Endnotes

1 - https://www.cdc.gov/obesity/data/adult.html

2 - https://pubmed.ncbi.nlm.nih.gov/29655062/